# DAMON REED

# HIIT

*Burn more fat in less time*

This book was professionally typeset on Reedsy.
Find out more at reedsy.com

# Contents

# 1

# Introduction

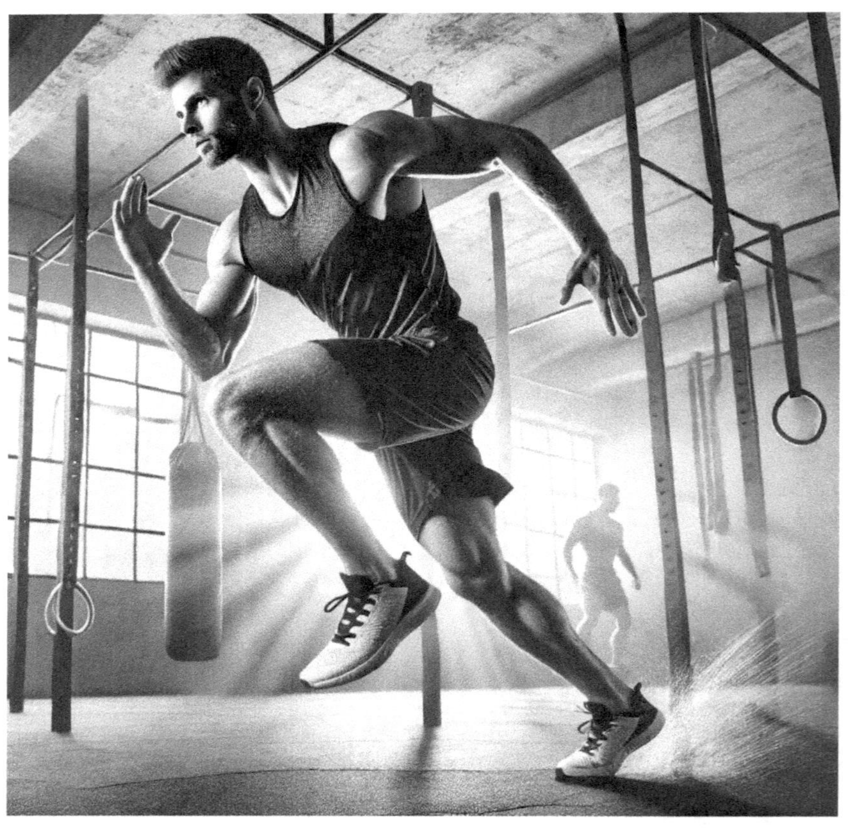

igh-Intensity Interval Training, or HIIT, is more than just another workout trend — it is a revolution in how we approach fitness. If you have ever struggled to find time for exercise, felt frustrated with workouts that seem to yield little progress, or wished there was a faster, smarter way to achieve your goals, HIIT might just be the solution you have been searching for. This book was created to give you everything you need to know about HIIT: how it works, why it's so effective, and how you can use it to burn fat, build endurance, and transform your body in less time than you thought possible.

Let's be honest — most of us lead busy lives. Between work, family, and personal commitments, finding an hour or two to dedicate to the gym can feel impossible. Even when we do carve out the time, traditional workouts can feel monotonous, and the results often come too slowly. HIIT changes all of that. By combining short bursts of intense effort with brief recovery periods, HIIT delivers maximum impact in minimal time. It's not just about working out harder; it's about working out smarter.

This book was born from my own journey of frustration with traditional fitness routines. Like many people, I struggled to balance a full schedule with the desire to stay fit. The breakthrough came when I discovered the science behind HIIT. Not only did it help me achieve better results in less time, but it also completely transformed the way I viewed exercise. I wrote this book to share that transformation with you and to empower you with a tool that can fit seamlessly into your life.

In the chapters ahead, we will dive deep into everything you need to know about HIIT. We will start by answering the fundamental question: what is HIIT? You will learn how it differs from traditional/continuous workouts, why it has gained so much popularity, and what makes it a game-changer for people with tight schedules. It certainly has been a game changer for me. Then, we will explore the science behind HIIT, breaking down how it burns fat, boosts metabolism, and continues working long after your workout is over — a phenomenon known as the "afterburn effect."

Once you understand the mechanics, we will get practical. You will learn how to design and implement HIIT workouts that fit your goals, whether you are looking to lose weight, build strength, or improve cardiovascular fitness. We will discuss how to structure your sessions, what duration and intensity to aim for, and how often you should train. For those new to fitness, we will cover beginner-friendly approaches, and for experienced athletes, we will offer advanced strategies to push your limits.

Of course, no workout program is without its risks. That is why we will also address the potential downsides of HIIT and how to avoid common pitfalls like overtraining or injury. By the end of this book, you will have a clear, actionable plan to make HIIT a sustainable and effective part of your fitness routine.

This book is not just about theory; it is about giving you the tools to act. Whether you're looking to lose a few pounds, improve your endurance, or simply make fitness fit into your life, HIIT has the potential to deliver life-changing results. The beauty of HIIT is its flexibility — it can be done at home or in the gym, with or without equipment, and adapted to suit any fitness level.

By the time you finish reading, you will not only understand what makes HIIT so powerful, but you will also be ready to put it into practice. You will have a clear roadmap for achieving your fitness goals in less time than you ever thought possible. More importantly, you will have the confidence to take control of your health and make lasting changes that fit your lifestyle.

So, are you ready to get started? In the next chapter, we will explore exactly what HIIT is and why it is one of the most effective workout methods ever developed. Let's dive in and discover how you can burn more fat in less time.

# 2

# What is HIIT?

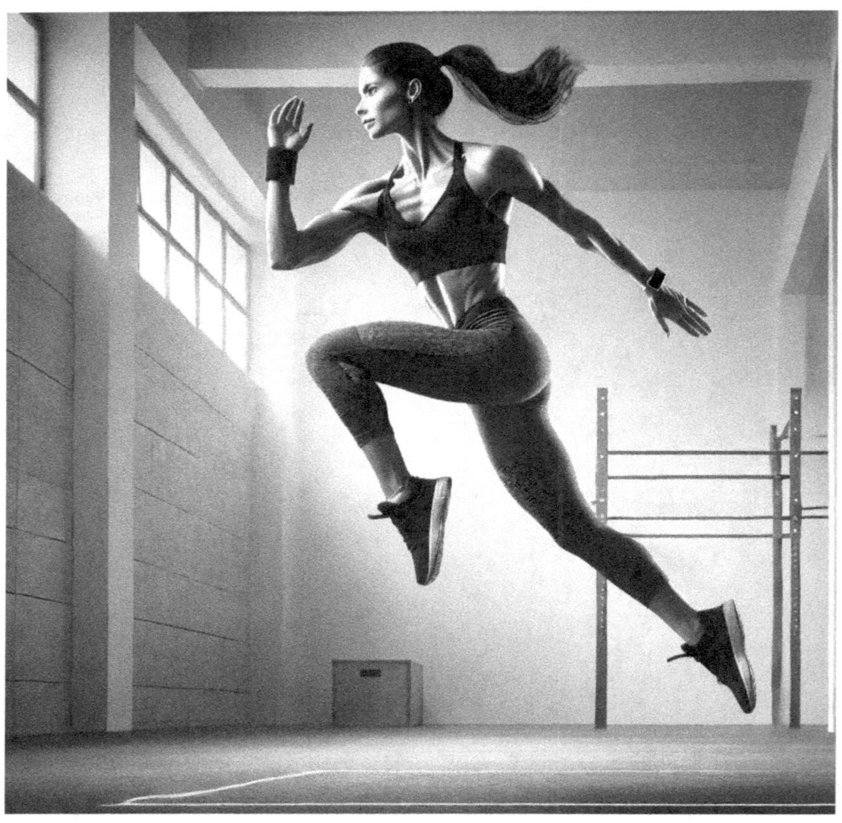

H IIT, or High-Intensity Interval Training, is a workout style built around alternating between periods of maximum effort and short recovery intervals. These intense bursts of activity push your body to its limits, while the rest periods allow just enough recovery to prepare for the next round. This structure keeps your heart rate elevated throughout the workout, which not only burns calories but also trains your cardiovascular system to work more efficiently.The term "high-intensity interval training" highlights its defining features: the **intensity** of effort during work phases and the **intervals** of rest that punctuate the workout. A classic HIIT session might involve 20 to 30 seconds of sprinting or jumping followed by 10 to 15 seconds of walking or resting, repeated in cycles for a total workout duration of 15 to 30 minutes. This unique format is what sets HIIT apart from traditional steady-state workouts, which often involve maintaining a moderate, consistent pace over a longer period.

## Who is it for?

HIIT is a versatile workout approach that caters to a wide range of fitness levels, lifestyles, and goals. It is especially appealing to those with busy schedules who struggle to find time for long workout sessions. With most HIIT routines lasting 15 to 30 minutes, it's an ideal solution for professionals, students, and parents looking for maximum results in minimal time. The flexibility of HIIT allows it to be performed anywhere—at the gym, at home, or even outdoors—making it accessible regardless of location or equipment availability.

While HIIT can be adapted for many age groups, it may not be suitable for everyone without adjustments. Seniors, for instance, can benefit from low-impact HIIT variations that focus on controlled movements and longer recovery periods. These modifications ensure that older adults can safely improve their cardiovascular health, endurance, and strength without overexerting themselves. However, seniors or individuals with pre-existing health conditions should always consult a healthcare professional or fitness expert before starting HIIT to ensure safety.

For younger individuals or those with a more active lifestyle, HIIT is an excellent way to add variety to workouts and break through fitness plateaus. It's also highly suitable for beginners, as workouts can be scaled to match their current fitness level and gradually increased in intensity as they progress. The customizable nature of HIIT makes it a practical option for almost anyone seeking an effective and time-efficient fitness routine, provided it's tailored to individual needs and abilities.

**Benefits of HIIT**

Incorporating HIIT into your everyday workouts offers a host of benefits, especially for those who value efficiency and effectiveness. One of the most significant advantages of HIIT is its ability to deliver **maximum results in minimal time**. Unlike traditional workouts, which often require 45 minutes to an hour of steady effort, HIIT sessions can be completed in as little as 15 to 30 minutes. This makes it an ideal solution for busy individuals who struggle to find time for longer workouts.

HIIT is also incredibly effective at burning calories and reducing fat, both during the workout and afterward. The high-intensity intervals push your body to work harder than it typically would, creating a phenomenon known as the **afterburn effect** (or excess post-exercise oxygen consumption, EPOC). This means your body continues to burn calories for hours after the workout ends, maximizing fat loss with less time spent exercising.

Beyond fat-burning, HIIT improves cardiovascular health by challenging your heart and lungs to operate at peak efficiency. It enhances oxygen consumption, lowers resting heart rate, and boosts overall endurance. Additionally, HIIT can be easily adapted to target specific goals, such as building strength, improving athletic performance, or losing weight.

Finally, HIIT's versatility makes it accessible and engaging. With endless combinations of exercises, intensities, and recovery periods, it ensures variety and helps prevent workout boredom. Whether you're performing sprints, bodyweight movements, or resistance exercises, HIIT keeps things fresh while delivering impressive results in a fraction of the time.

**Difference Between HIIT and Traditional Workouts**

HIIT and traditional workouts differ significantly in structure, intensity, and outcomes. HIIT alternates between short bursts of maximum-effort exercise and brief recovery periods, typically lasting 15 to 30 minutes. In contrast, traditional workouts often involve steady, moderate-intensity effort maintained over a longer duration, such as 45 to 60 minutes of jogging, cycling, or weightlifting.

Here's how they compare:
  **Time Efficiency:**

- HIIT: Designed for busy individuals, HIIT delivers comparable—or even superior—results in less time, with most sessions lasting 15 to 30 minutes.
- Traditional Workouts: These require more time, typically lasting 45 to 60 minutes, to achieve similar results.

**Calorie Burn and Afterburn Effect:**

- HIIT: Burns more calories during the workout and triggers the "afterburn effect" (excess post-exercise oxygen consumption, or EPOC), causing your body to burn additional calories for hours post-exercise.
- Traditional Workouts: Calorie burn is limited to the workout duration, with little to no afterburn effect.

**Intensity and Variability:**

- HIIT: Alternates between intense bursts of activity and recovery, keeping the body challenged and engaged.
- Traditional Workouts: Emphasizes consistent, moderate effort over a longer duration, often at a steady pace.

**Customizability:**

- HIIT: Easily adjustable to suit all fitness levels and goals. You can modify the exercises, intervals, and intensity to meet your specific needs.
- Traditional Workouts: Require more time and a higher baseline fitness level to see significant benefits, and they are generally less adaptable to time constraints.

In summary, HIIT offers a more efficient, versatile, and dynamic approach to fitness compared to traditional workouts. Whether your goal is fat loss, endurance, or overall health, HIIT provides a flexible and engaging alternative that fits into even the busiest of schedules.

# 3

# The Science Behind HIIT

The effectiveness of HIIT lies in the physiological responses it triggers during and after the workout. By alternating short bursts of maximum effort with brief recovery periods, HIIT delivers a unique combination of cardiovascular, metabolic, and muscular benefits that traditional workouts often can't match.

For cardiovascular fitness, HIIT pushes the heart and lungs to operate at peak capacity during intense intervals, which improves oxygen delivery and utilization. This strengthens the cardiovascular system and increases VO2 max, a key measure of aerobic fitness. Unlike steady-state cardio, HIIT simultaneously trains the anaerobic system, building the ability to perform short, explosive efforts while enhancing long-term stamina.

HIIT is also highly effective for weight loss. Its high-intensity structure activates fat-burning hormones and boosts metabolism, with the added benefit of the "afterburn effect." This phenomenon, known as excess post-exercise oxygen consumption (EPOC), causes the body to continue burning calories long after the workout ends, making HIIT particularly efficient for reducing fat.

The benefits of HIIT extend beyond fitness and weight loss. It improves sleep quality by reducing stress and regulating circadian rhythms, promoting deeper, more restorative rest. Better sleep enhances recovery and energy levels, creating a positive feedback loop for maintaining an active lifestyle.

HIIT also supports muscle growth and preservation. Unlike traditional cardio, which can sometimes lead to muscle loss, HIIT incorporates movements that challenge muscles, such as squats, lunges, and push-ups. These exercises build strength and lean mass, making it an ideal choice for improving overall body composition.The science behind HIIT explains its unparalleled efficiency.  By engaging both aerobic and anaerobic systems, optimizing fat loss, improving sleep, and building muscle, HIIT offers a comprehensive approach to fitness that is as time efficient as it is effective.

**Fat/Weight Loss**

HIIT is one of the most effective workout methods for fat loss, and the science behind its success explains why it has become so popular. By alternating between intense bursts of activity and short recovery periods, HIIT pushes the body to its metabolic limits, forcing it to burn more calories during the workout and well after it ends.  This unique combination of high-intensity effort and recovery creates an optimal environment for fat-burning that few other workout styles can match.

A key component of HIIT's fat-loss power is the **afterburn effect**, formally known as excess post-exercise oxygen consumption (EPOC).

During a HIIT session:

- The body operates at near-maximal capacity, creating an oxygen deficit.
- After the workout, the body works overtime to replenish oxygen, repair muscle tissue, and remove metabolic byproducts like lactic acid.
- These recovery processes require significant energy, keeping your metabolism elevated for hours—sometimes up to 24 hours—after the workout.This extended calorie burn makes HIIT particularly effective for reducing body fat, including stubborn areas like the abdomen.

HIIT also improves **VO2 max**, a measure of the maximum amount of oxygen the body can utilize during exercise.

A higher VO2 max translates to:

- The ability to perform more intense and prolonged physical activity, increasing overall calorie burn.
- Enhanced aerobic efficiency, enabling the body to access and burn fat more effectively as an energy source.This dual action—training both the aerobic and anaerobic systems—makes HIIT a powerful tool for fat loss.

What sets HIIT apart from traditional cardio workouts is its ability to target **visceral fat**, the fat stored around internal organs. Research shows that HIIT is more effective than steady-state cardio at reducing visceral fat.

This is because:

- HIIT stimulates fat-burning hormones, such as epinephrine and

norepinephrine, which mobilize stored fat for energy.
- The intense intervals force the body to prioritize fat as a fuel source during recovery.

Additionally, HIIT's ability to **preserve or build muscle mass** while reducing fat gives it a distinct edge. Many HIIT workouts incorporate resistance-based exercises, such as:

- Squats
- Push-ups
- Kettlebell swingsThese movements help build strength and maintain lean muscle, ensuring the weight lost through HIIT is primarily fat, resulting in a more defined and toned body composition.

In conclusion, HIIT's combination of the afterburn effect, VO2 max improvements, hormone activation, and its ability to fit into even the busiest of schedules makes it one of the most effective and efficient workouts for fat loss. By targeting stubborn fat areas, enhancing metabolism, and preserving lean muscle, HIIT provides a comprehensive and sustainable approach to achieving your weight-loss goals.

**Muscle Building**

Unlike traditional cardio, which can sometimes lead to muscle loss due to prolonged energy expenditure, HIIT is uniquely effective at preserving and even building muscle while simultaneously burning fat. The secret lies in the structure of HIIT workouts and how they challenge both the cardiovascular and muscular systems simultaneously.

HIIT often incorporates resistance-based movements such as squats, lunges, push-ups, and kettlebell swings. These exercises engage multiple muscle groups and create the necessary stimulus for muscle growth. The high-intensity nature of these movements forces the muscles to work harder in a short amount of time, mimicking the effects of traditional strength training. Over time, this leads to increased muscle mass and improved muscle definition.

Additionally, HIIT triggers the release of growth-promoting hormones like testosterone and human growth hormone (HGH), which play a crucial role in muscle repair and growth. The alternating bursts of effort and recovery periods also reduce the risk of muscle fatigue associated with prolonged steady-state cardio, preserving lean muscle mass.

One of HIIT's greatest advantages is its ability to simultaneously burn fat while maintaining or building muscle. This dual effect results in a more toned and defined physique. As fat decreases and muscle density increases, the body appears leaner, stronger, and more athletic. Incorporating HIIT into your routine not only enhances muscle strength but also improves functional fitness, making everyday activities easier and more efficient.

Over time, regular HIIT workouts transform your body composition, shifting the focus from simply losing weight to building a leaner, more muscular frame. This comprehensive approach makes HIIT a valuable addition to any fitness plan, whether your goal is to build muscle, burn fat, or achieve a balanced and toned physique.

**Anaerobic and Aerobic Systems**

HIIT is unique in its ability to simultaneously challenge and improve both the anaerobic and aerobic energy systems, creating a well-rounded and highly effective workout. Each system is responsible for providing energy under different conditions, and HIIT's alternating periods of high-intensity effort and recovery engage both systems in a dynamic way.

**Anaerobic System**

The anaerobic system is activated during the intense bursts of a HIIT workout when the body needs immediate energy to sustain high effort. This system generates energy without relying on oxygen, instead using glycogen stored in the muscles. This is critical for powering short, explosive movements such as sprints, jumps, or heavy resistance exercises.

HIIT enhances the anaerobic system by improving the body's ability to tolerate and clear lactic acid, a byproduct of anaerobic activity. Over time, this reduces muscle fatigue during high-intensity efforts and increases your capacity for short bursts of power. By repeatedly engaging the anaerobic system in a controlled and structured way, HIIT trains the body to recover more efficiently between intense efforts, improving performance in sports, strength training, and other physically demanding activities.

**Aerobic System**

The aerobic system, in contrast, provides energy during lower-intensity, sustained activities and recovery periods. It relies on oxygen to break down carbohydrates and fat into usable energy, making it the primary energy source during HIIT's recovery intervals. As you recover between high-intensity bursts, the aerobic system replenishes energy stores and clears waste products like lactic acid, preparing the body for the next round of effort.

Regular HIIT training strengthens the aerobic system by improving oxygen delivery and utilization. This increases cardiovascular efficiency, enhancing endurance and stamina. The aerobic benefits of HIIT are comparable to those of traditional steady-state cardio, but they are achieved in a fraction of the time due to the workout's intensity and structure.

**How HIIT Balances Both Systems**

HIIT's unique design—alternating between high-intensity intervals that activate the anaerobic system and recovery periods that engage the aerobic system—creates a powerful synergy. This dual training improves both short-term power and long-term endurance. Over time, the body becomes more efficient at switching between these systems, resulting in:

- Enhanced athletic performance
- Faster recovery during physical activities
- Greater stamina for sustained efforts
- Improved metabolic flexibility, or the ability to efficiently use both carbohydrates and fat as energy sources

By engaging both the anaerobic and aerobic systems, HIIT provides a comprehensive workout that not only boosts cardiovascular and muscular performance but also maximizes calorie burn and overall fitness. This balanced development makes it a versatile and effective method for improving multiple aspects of physical health.

**The effect on sleep**

HIIT not only improves physical fitness but also has a significant positive impact on sleep quality. The intense physical exertion during a HIIT workout promotes better sleep by helping to regulate the body's natural circadian rhythms, which control the sleep-wake cycle. Engaging in regular HIIT sessions can enhance your ability to fall asleep faster and experience deeper, more restorative sleep.

One way HIIT influences sleep is through its ability to reduce stress and anxiety. The high-intensity nature of the workout releases endorphins, which are natural mood elevators that help reduce stress levels. Lower stress allows the mind and body to relax, making it easier to wind down at night. Additionally, HIIT helps reduce levels of cortisol, the stress hormone that can interfere with sleep when chronically elevated.

HIIT also physically tires the body in a productive way, encouraging it to seek recovery through sleep. The energy expenditure and muscle repair needed after a high-intensity session make the body more inclined to enter the deeper stages of sleep, such as REM (rapid eye movement) and slow-wave sleep, both of which are critical for recovery and overall health. These stages are when the body repairs muscle tissue, consolidates memories, and restores energy.

Timing, however, is key. Performing HIIT too close to bedtime can sometimes have the opposite effect, as the adrenaline and elevated heart rate from the workout might make it harder to fall asleep immediately. It's best to schedule HIIT sessions earlier in the day or at least a few hours before bedtime to fully reap the sleep-enhancing benefits.

By improving the quality and duration of sleep, HIIT supports recovery, boosts energy levels, and enhances overall well-being. Better sleep also creates a positive feedback loop, allowing for more effective workouts and greater consistency in your fitness routine. Incorporating HIIT into your lifestyle can thus lead to a cycle of improved fitness, reduced stress, and optimal sleep health.

4

# HIIT - Implementation

HIIT is one of the most adaptable workout formats, making it suitable for a range of fitness goals and exercise styles. This chapter explores how HIIT can be incorporated into different workout types, offering targeted benefits such as weight loss, improved cardiovascular fitness, enhanced cross-training performance, and strength building. To help you get started, each section also provides practical sample exercises.

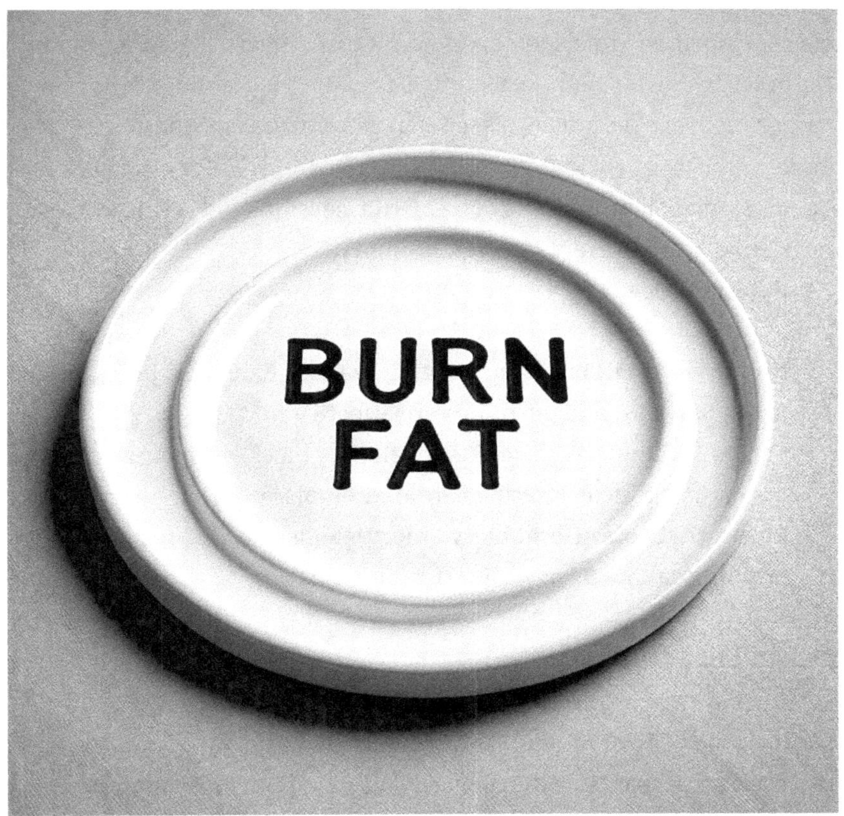



**HIIT and Fat/Weight Loss**

HIIT is one of the most effective methods for fat loss because it maximizes calorie burn in a short time and triggers the afterburn effect,
where your body continues burning calories even after the workout ends.
Incorporating HIIT into a fat-loss plan requires a balance of consistent
exercise, proper nutrition, and a realistic approach to achieving results.

**How to Incorporate HIIT for Fat Loss**

To start, choose exercises that elevate your heart rate quickly, such as burpees, sprints, jump squats, or mountain climbers. Beginners should begin with shorter high-intensity intervals (20 seconds) followed by longer recovery periods (40 seconds). Over time as fitness improves, increase the length of high-intensity intervals and reduce recovery times. Consistency is key, so aim for 3-4 HIIT sessions per week, ensuring recovery days to prevent burnout or injury.

### Equipment Needed

- **Bodyweight HIIT:** No equipment needed. Exercises like jumping jacks, burpees, and push-ups are effective for fat loss.
- **Cardio Machines:** Treadmills, stationary bikes, or rowing machines are great for incorporating cardio intervals.
- **Strength Tools:** Dumbbells or kettlebells can add resistance, increasing calorie burn while engaging muscles.

## The Role of Nutrition

Exercise alone isn't enough to achieve significant fat loss—nutrition plays a critical role. A well-balanced diet fuels your workouts, supports recovery, and helps create the calorie deficit necessary for fat loss. Focus on:

- **Lean Proteins:** Chicken, fish, tofu, or legumes to support muscle repair and growth.
- **Complex Carbohydrates:** Brown rice, quinoa, or sweet potatoes for sustained energy.
- **Healthy Fats:** Avocados, nuts, or olive oil to support overall health.
- **Vegetables and Fruits:** Rich in vitamins, minerals, and fiber for digestion and satiety.Avoid overly restrictive diets, as they can lead to fatigue, muscle loss, and inconsistency. Instead, aim for sustainable changes that align with your lifestyle.

**Sample HIIT Workout for Fat Loss**

This workout combines cardio and bodyweight exercises to maximize calorie burn:

1. **Jump squats:** 30 seconds at maximum effort
2. **Rest:** 15 seconds
3. **Burpees:** 30 seconds
4. **Rest:** 15 seconds
5. **High knees:** 30 seconds
6. **Rest:** 15 seconds
7. **Mountain climbers:** 30 seconds
8. **Rest:** 30 secondsRepeat the cycle 3-4 times, depending on your fitness level.

**Progression Tips**

- Gradually increase the intensity or reduce rest periods as your fitness improves.
- Incorporate resistance exercises like kettlebell swings or dumbbell thrusters to challenge muscles and burn more calories.
- Monitor your nutrition and adjust as needed to maintain a calorie deficit while staying energized for workouts.

By combining HIIT with a balanced diet and proper recovery, you can achieve fat loss effectively and sustainably. HIIT not only burns fat but also improves cardiovascular fitness and preserves lean muscle, leading to a leaner, stronger, and healthier physique.

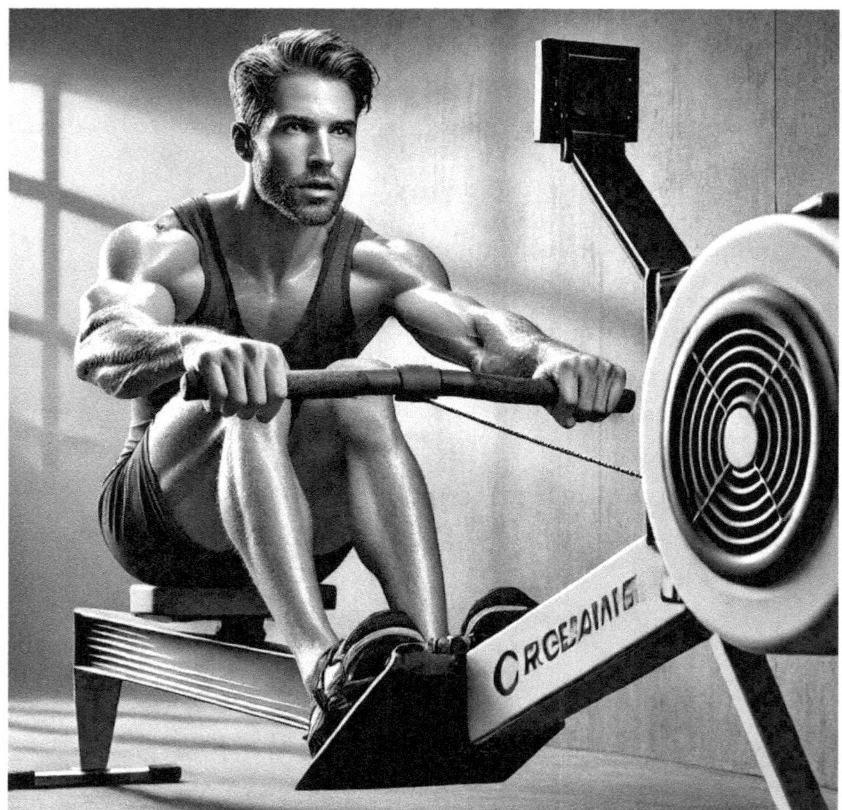


## HIIT and Cardio

Incorporating cardio into HIIT is a powerful way to improve cardiovascular fitness, burn calories, and enhance endurance. Unlike traditional steady-state cardio, such as jogging or cycling at a constant pace, HIIT cardio alternates between short bursts of maximum effort and recovery periods. This approach keeps your heart rate elevated, challenges your cardiovascular system, and maximizes calorie burn in a shorter time.

To start, choose a cardio activity that you enjoy and that aligns with your fitness level. Popular options include running, cycling, rowing, or using equipment like an elliptical machine. Beginners should begin with shorter high-intensity intervals and longer recovery periods—for example, 20 seconds of intense effort followed by 40 seconds of slow-paced recovery. As your fitness improves, you can increase the intensity, reduce the recovery time, or extend the duration of the high-intensity intervals.

**Equipment Needed:**

- **For Running:** A safe, flat space like a track or treadmill.
- **For Cycling:** A stationary bike or outdoor bicycle.
- **For Rowing:** A rowing machine is ideal.
- **Bodyweight Cardio:** No equipment is necessary; moves like jumping jacks, high knees, and burpees can also be incorporated.

When incorporating cardio into HIIT, it's important to warm up properly to prepare your body for the high-intensity effort. A 5-10 minute warm-up of light jogging, dynamic stretches, or cycling at a moderate pace will help reduce the risk of injury and improve performance.

**Sample Cardio HIIT Workout (Running):**

- Warm-up: 5 minutes of light jogging
- Sprint: 20 seconds at maximum effort
- Walk or jog: 40 seconds at a comfortable pace
- Repeat for 10-15 minutes
- Cool down: 5 minutes of walking or slow jogging

This simple yet effective structure can also be adapted for other forms of cardio, such as cycling or rowing. For example, on a stationary bike, you might alternate between 20 seconds of pedaling as fast as possible and 40 seconds of slow, easy pedaling.

Incorporating cardio into HIIT sessions offers an efficient way to build endurance, improve heart health, and burn calories in a short amount of time. With consistency and progression, this approach will help you achieve your fitness goals while keeping your workouts dynamic and engaging.

**HIIT and Cross-Training**

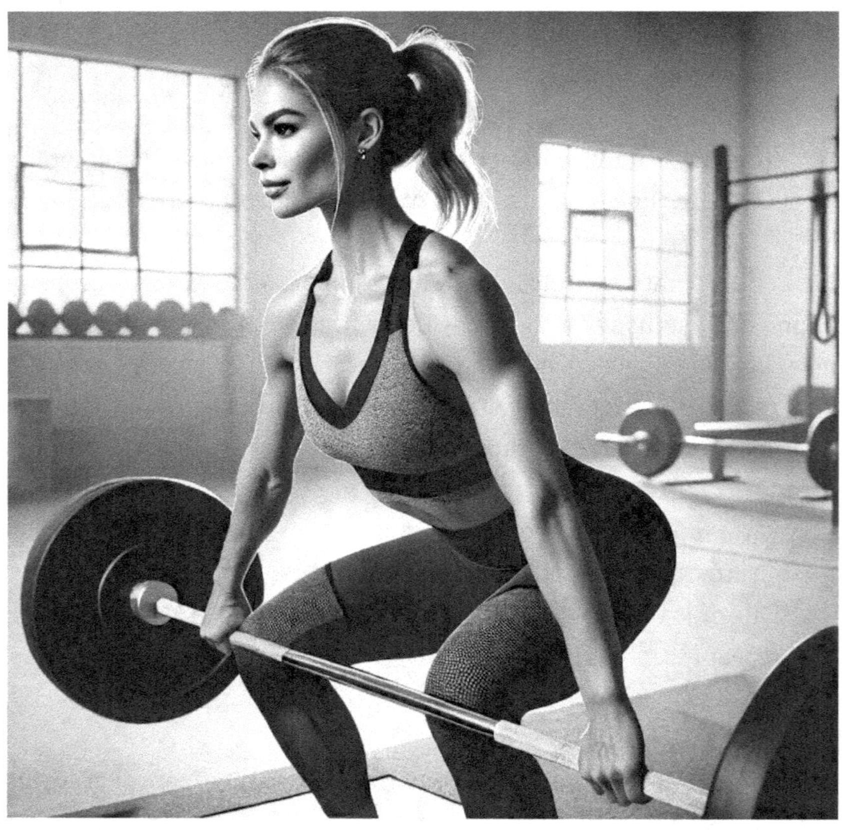

**HIIT and Cross-Training**

Incorporating cross-training into HIIT is an excellent way to boost overall fitness, improve athletic performance, and prevent workout monotony. Cross-training combines different types of exercises—such as running, cycling, strength training, and bodyweight movements—targeting multiple muscle groups and fitness components. Adding a HIIT structure to cross-training introduces intensity and variety, enhancing the workout's effectiveness.

## How to Incorporate Cross-Training into HIIT

To start, identify the main activities in your cross-training routine and select exercises that complement one another. For example, combine cardio (like running or cycling) with functional strength exercises (such as kettlebell swings or lunges) to create a balanced and engaging workout. Start with shorter intervals of high-intensity effort (20-30 seconds) and longer recovery periods (30-60 seconds). As you gain fitness, increase the intensity or reduce the recovery time.

### Equipment Needed

- **For Cardio Elements:** Treadmill, stationary bike, rowing machine, or an outdoor space for sprints.
- **For Strength and Bodyweight Moves:** Kettlebells, dumbbells, or resistance bands for added resistance.
- **For Functional Movements:** A jump rope, plyo box, or medicine ball to add variety and challenge.

## Sample HIIT Cross-Training Workout

This sample combines cardio, strength, and functional movements into a high-intensity cross-training session:

1.  **Rowing (or cycling):** 30 seconds at maximum effort
2.  **Rest:** 15 seconds
3.  **Kettlebell swings:** 30 seconds
4.  **Rest:** 15 seconds
5.  **Burpees:** 30 seconds
6.  **Rest:** 15 seconds
7.  **Box jumps:** 30 seconds
8.  **Rest:** 30 secondsRepeat this cycle 3-4 times, depending on your fitness level.

**Progression Tips**

- Beginners should prioritize proper form and use lighter weights or lower-impact variations (e.g., step-ups instead of box jumps).
- Gradually increase intensity by reducing recovery time, increasing weight, or adding more challenging movements as your fitness improves.
- Incorporate a variety of exercises to target different muscle groups and maintain workout engagement.

Cross-training in a HIIT format delivers a comprehensive workout that enhances endurance, strength, agility, and coordination. This approach not only improves overall athleticism but also keeps workouts fresh and exciting, making it easier to stay consistent and achieve your fitness goals.

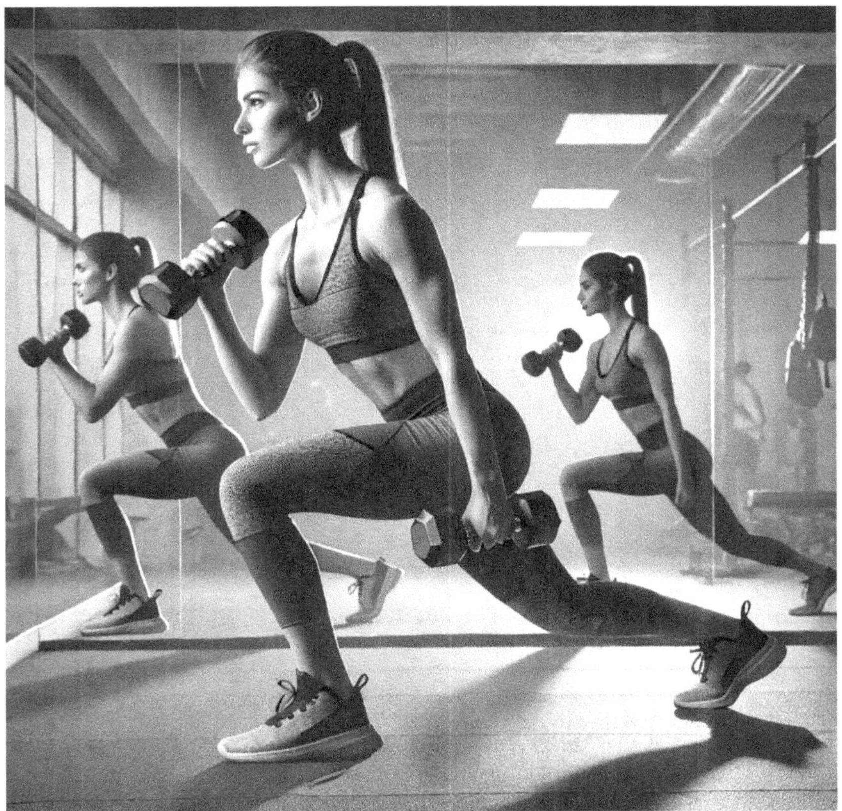

## HIIT and Weightlifting

Combining HIIT with weightlifting is a powerful way to build muscle, improve strength, and burn fat simultaneously. By incorporating resistance exercises into a HIIT structure, you can elevate your heart rate while engaging multiple muscle groups. This approach not only maximizes calorie burn but also enhances muscular endurance and promotes lean muscle growth, making it ideal for those looking to improve body composition.

## How to Start

To begin, focus on compound movements like squats, deadlifts, or kettlebell swings, which work several muscle groups at once. Beginners should start with lighter weights to ensure proper form during high-intensity intervals and gradually increase resistance as their strength improves. A typical HIIT and weight-lifting workout alternates between a weighted exercise and a short recovery period, with 20-30 seconds of effort followed by 20-40 seconds of rest. Aim for 3-4 sessions per week to allow for recovery and muscle growth.

**Equipment Needed**

- Dumbbells, kettlebells, or barbells for weighted movements
- A workout bench or stability ball for exercises like bench presses or supported rows
- Resistance bands for added variety and portability
- An open space to safely perform dynamic movements like weighted lunges or kettlebell swings

**Sample HIIT and Weightlifting Workout**

This workout targets strength and endurance, alternating between resistance exercises and short recovery periods:

1. **Kettlebell swings:** 30 seconds
2. **Rest:** 15 seconds
3. **Weighted squats (use dumbbells or a barbell):** 30 seconds
4. **Rest:** 15 seconds
5. **Push press (dumbbell or barbell):** 30 seconds
6. **Rest:** 15 seconds
7. **Renegade rows (dumbbells):** 30 seconds
8. **Rest:** 30 secondsRepeat this cycle 3-4 times, depending on your fitness level.

## Progression Tips

- Beginners should focus on mastering form and control during each movement to prevent injury.
- Gradually increase weight or reduce rest periods to make the workout more challenging as you progress.
- Incorporate new movements, such as deadlifts, clean-and-presses, or lunges, to target different muscle groups and keep workouts engaging.

By blending HIIT with weight lifting, you achieve a dual-action workout that builds strength and burns calories efficiently. This approach ensures you preserve and develop muscle mass while enhancing cardiovascular fitness, making it a comprehensive solution for those aiming to sculpt a lean and powerful physique.

5

# HIIT Risk

igh-Intensity Interval Training (HIIT) is an incredibly effective workout method, but like any form of exercise, it comes with its own set of risks—especially if overdone or performed incorrectly. Understanding these risks and learning how to prevent them is essential for safely incorporating HIIT into your fitness routine. This chapter explores the potential dangers of HIIT, how to mitigate them, and how to determine if HIIT is the right workout for you.

**The Risks of Overdoing HIIT**

HIIT's demanding nature can lead to several risks if not properly managed:

1. **Overtraining:** Too many HIIT sessions without sufficient recovery can lead to fatigue, decreased performance, and even injuries. The body needs time to repair muscle fibers and replenish energy stores, making rest days crucial.
2. **Injury Risk:** The explosive movements and high-impact exercises

in HIIT, such as jump squats or burpees, can put stress on joints, muscles, and tendons, increasing the likelihood of strains, sprains, or other injuries.

3. **Cardiovascular Strain:** For individuals with pre-existing heart conditions or those who are new to exercise, the intensity of HIIT may put excessive strain on the heart and cardiovascular system.

4. **Burnout:** The mental and physical demands of HIIT can lead to burnout if workouts are too frequent or intense, reducing motivation and consistency over time.

## How to Manage Risks

To minimize the risks associated with HIIT, follow these guidelines:

- **Prioritize Recovery:** Schedule at least one to two rest or low-intensity days per week to allow your body to recover and adapt.
- **Warm-Up and Cool Down:** Properly warming up prepares your body for intense activity, while cooling down reduces soreness and aids recovery.
- **Focus on Form:** Ensure you have mastered the correct technique for each movement before increasing intensity to avoid injury.
- **Start Slowly:** Beginners should start with shorter intervals and longer recovery periods, gradually increasing intensity as fitness improves.
- **Listen to Your Body:** Pay attention to signs of overtraining, such as persistent fatigue, pain, or a lack of progress. Adjust your routine as needed.

## Is HIIT Suitable for You?

While HIIT is an excellent workout for many, it may not be suitable for everyone. Consider the following factors before starting:

- **Fitness Level:** Beginners should ease into HIIT gradually, ensuring they have a baseline level of fitness.
- **Health Conditions:** Individuals with heart problems, joint issues, or other medical concerns should consult a healthcare provider before starting HIIT.
- **Personal Goals:** HIIT is ideal for improving cardiovascular fitness, burning fat, and building endurance, but it may not align with goals that require low-intensity or long-duration exercise.

HIIT is highly effective but requires careful execution to minimize risks. By understanding potential dangers, prioritizing recovery, and tailoring workouts to your fitness level, you can safely enjoy its benefits. Assess your health and readiness to determine if HIIT suits your goals, and with the right precautions, it can be a transformative tool in your fitness journey.

# 6

# Conclusion

**H**IIT is more than just a workout trend—it's a proven, science-backed approach to achieving remarkable fitness results in a fraction of the time. From improving cardiovascular health to burning fat, building muscle, and enhancing endurance, HIIT offers a comprehensive solution for a wide range of fitness goals. Its versatility allows it to be adapted to suit any fitness level, lifestyle, or objective, making it accessible to everyone, from beginners to elite athletes.

Throughout this book, we've explored the many facets of HIIT, from its scientific principles to practical implementation. You've learned how HIIT can revolutionize your fitness routine, whether through cardio, weightlifting, cross-training, or fat loss-focused sessions. We've also discussed how to safely incorporate HIIT, emphasizing the importance of recovery, proper nutrition, and listening to your body to avoid burnout or injury.

Now is the time to take action. Whether you're just starting your fitness journey or looking to elevate your current routine, HIIT provides the tools you need to succeed. Begin with a plan that aligns with your goals, stay consistent, and track your progress. Remember, the key to long-term success is balancing effort with recovery and maintaining a sustainable approach to your workouts and overall health.

As you embark on your HIIT journey, I hope this book has inspired you to take charge of your fitness in a way that is efficient, effective, and empowering. Your feedback is incredibly valuable—not just to me but to others who may benefit from this guide. If you found this book helpful, I'd greatly appreciate it if you could take a moment to leave a review on Amazon. Your insights can help others discover the transformative potential of HIIT.

Here's to your success and a healthier, stronger you. Let the power of HIIT propel you toward your goals!

# 7

# Resources

Atakan, M. M., Li, Y., Koşar, Ş. N., Turnagöl, H. H., & Yan, X. (2021). Evidence-Based Effects of High-Intensity Interval Training on Exercise Capacity and Health: A Review with Historical Perspective. *International Journal of Environmental Research and Public Health*, *18*(13), 7201. https://doi.org/10.3390/ijerph18137201

*The Science Behind HIIT Workouts.* (2017, July 11). St. Luke's Health. https://www.stlukeshealth.org/resources/science-behind-hiit-workouts

Stiehl, B. C. (2024, August 14). The Science Behind HIIT Afterburn Effect. *Shape.* https://www.shape.com/fitness/tips/science-behind-afterburn-effect

Millar, J. (n.d.). *HIIT is changing the way we work out, here's the science why it works.* https://www.sciencefocus.com/the-human-body/hiit-is-changing-the-way-we-workout-heres-the-science-why-it-works

*The Science Behind High Intensity Interval Training (HIIT) | Cornerstone Health & Fitness.* (2024, September 16). Cornerstone Health & Fitness | Best Gym in Bucks County Pennsylvania. https://cornerstoneclubs.com/gym-news/the-science-behind-high-intensity-interval-training-hiit/

Liam. (2024, January 14). *High-Intensity Interval Training(HIIT) and Its Impact on Sleep.* PhuketFit - Weight Loss & Fitness Retreat. https://phuketfit.com/high-intensity-interval-traininghiit-and-its-impact-on-sleep/

Online, C., & Online, C. (2020, February 2). *Ultimate Guide: High Intensity Interval Training (HIIT) For Weight Loss and Fat Loss.* Cardio Online Superstore. https://cardioonline.com.au/blogs/expert-advice/ultimate-guide-to-high-intensity-interval-training-hiit-for-weight-loss?srsltid=AfmBOoqkJYLSXWlU7ANZbPE0R2utzzeQRt2p3HLIIa6EdXuDAW34F1RZ

OpenAI. (2021). ChatGPT (GPT-4) [Software]. OpenAI. https://www.openai.com/

9 798302 749482